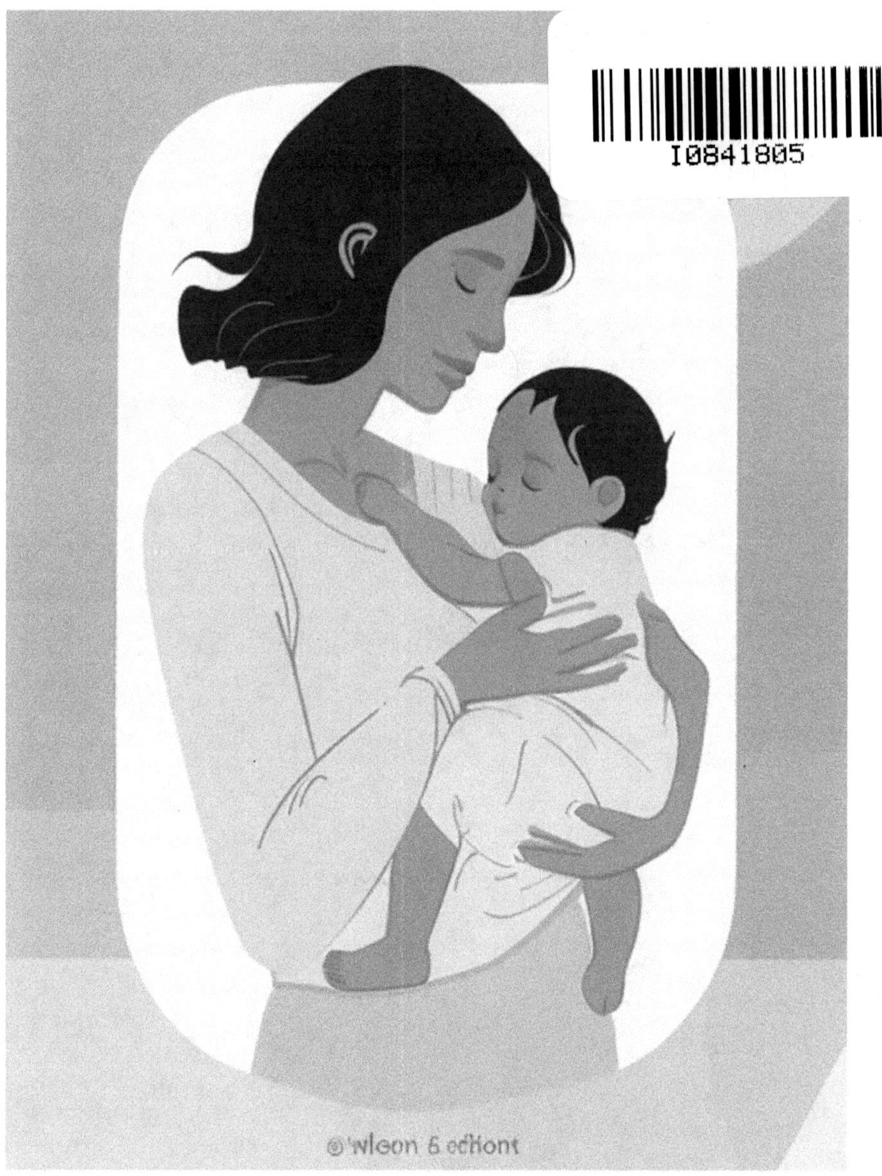

NURTURING MOM

A Guide to Managing Anxiety,
Rediscovering Identity,

and Embracing the Journey
of Motherhood

By:

Aisha Brady, LMSW-PMH

AISHA BRADY LMSW

Table of Contents

Intro

Embracing Motherhood: Nurturing Your Mental and Emotional Well-being

Motherhood is a remarkable journey that brings immense joy, love, and fulfillment into our lives. As moms, we dedicate ourselves to the well-being and happiness of our children, often putting their needs before our own. However, it's crucial to remember that our own mental and emotional well-being deserves equal attention and care. This book, "Embracing Motherhood: Nurturing Your Mental and Emotional Well-being," is designed to support and empower moms like you in navigating the complex terrain of motherhood while prioritizing your mental health.

In this comprehensive guide, we will tackle key topics that often impact moms, such as anxiety and depression. We will shed light on the common signs and symptoms that often go unnoticed, empowering you to recognize and address these challenges head-on. We will explore natural coping skills, self-care practices, and the importance of seeking professional help when necessary, ensuring you have a comprehensive toolkit to navigate the ups and downs of motherhood.

Additionally, we will discuss the fascinating correlation between women's mental health and physical health problems, emphasizing the need to prioritize self-care and mental well-being for overall health. Through my professional insights and personal experiences as a mother myself, you will gain a deeper understanding of the interconnectedness between mind and body, inspiring you to take proactive steps in nurturing both.

As you progress through this Book, you will find thought provoking reflections, and actionable tips that you can easily incorporate into your daily life. Whether you're a new mom, experienced mother, or navigating the challenges of different stages of motherhood, this book is tailored to meet your unique needs, providing guidance and support along the way.

Remember, taking care of yourself is not a luxury but a necessity. By investing in your mental and emotional well-being, you not only create a positive impact on yourself but also create a nurturing environment for your children and loved ones. Let this book be your companion on this transformative journey, empowering you to embrace motherhood with strength, resilience, and joy. Together, let us embark on a path of self-discovery, self-care, and empowerment, as we celebrate the incredible journey of motherhood and prioritize our mental and emotional well-being.

Chapter 1

Balancing Motherhood: Lessons from an Experienced Mom

As an experienced Licensed Master of Social Work (LMSW) and a Perinatal Mental Health Specialist (PMH); in addition to being a mother of three boys, and a survivor of postpartum depression and anxiety, I intimately understand the unique struggles that moms face in balancing the demands of motherhood with their own well-being. In this chapter, I will share my personal journey, which includes having my children within a five-year span, managing adult ADHD, and the impact it had on my marriage. Through my experiences, I hope to offer insights and guidance on how to navigate the challenges of motherhood while prioritizing self-care.

The Balancing Act of Motherhood

Motherhood is a beautiful and transformative experience, but it also comes with its fair share of challenges. Having three children in a short period meant that my life became a constant juggle of responsibilities, from diaper changes and feeding schedules to school activities and sleepless nights. The struggle to find balance between meeting the needs of my children, maintaining a household, and nurturing my own well-being was real. Here are a few ways I learned to manage the chaos.

1. Embracing Imperfection: One of the key lessons I learned early on was to embrace imperfection. It's impossible to be a perfect mother, and striving for perfection only adds unnecessary pressure. Accepting that there will be good days and challenging days

allowed me to let go of unrealistic expectations and focus on doing my best.

2. Setting Realistic Expectations: Recognizing my limitations and setting realistic expectations was essential. It meant being mindful of my energy levels and acknowledging that I couldn't do it all. By prioritizing tasks and seeking support when needed, I was able to navigate the overwhelming demands of motherhood more effectively.

3. Self-care often takes a backseat when we become mothers, as our focus naturally shifts towards our children. However, neglecting self-care can lead to burnout and negatively impact our mental and emotional well-being. It took time, but I learned the importance of self-care and developed strategies to incorporate it into my daily life.

4. Carving Out "Me" Time: Finding small pockets of time for myself became a priority. Whether it was waking up a few minutes earlier to enjoy a cup of coffee or tea, indulging in a hobby, or simply taking a walk alone, these moments of solitude rejuvenated me and helped me reconnect with myself.

5. Seeking Support: Recognizing the need for support and reaching out to others was a significant turning point for me. Whether it was asking for help from family and friends or joining a support group for moms, having a strong support network made a tremendous difference in my well-being.

Nurturing Marriage: Weathering the Storms of Parenthood

Marriage is a beautiful partnership that requires continuous effort and understanding, especially when children enter the picture. The arrival of children can bring immense joy, but it also introduces new dynamics and challenges to a marriage. Balancing the needs of children, household responsibilities, and personal well-being can strain even the strongest relationships. I personally experienced the following challenges:

1. Shifting Priorities: As mothers, our priorities naturally shift towards our children's well-being, which can inadvertently result in neglecting our partners. It's crucial to recognize and address this shift to maintain a healthy balance in the relationship.
2. Communication and Emotional Connection: The demands of parenthood can often leave little time for meaningful communication and emotional connection with our partners. I realized the importance of open and honest communication, finding quality time together, and expressing gratitude and appreciation.

Strategies for Maintaining a Strong Marriage

1. Date Nights and Quality Time: Carving out dedicated time for my partner became a priority. Regular date nights, even if they were simple and low-key, allowed us to reconnect and enjoy each other's company. Additionally, finding moments for quality time amidst the chaos of parenting reinforced our bond.
2. Shared Responsibilities: Sharing household and parenting responsibilities created a sense of partnership and equity within our marriage. By acknowledging and respecting each other's contributions, we were able to alleviate stress and maintain a more harmonious environment.

As moms, finding balance between motherhood and personal well-being is an ongoing journey. By acknowledging the challenges, embracing self-care, and nurturing our relationships, we can navigate the complexities of motherhood while maintaining our own happiness and fostering a thriving marriage. Remember, you are not alone in this journey, and by prioritizing yourself and your relationships, you can navigate the challenges of motherhood with resilience and love.

Chapter 2

Finding Your Identity
Amidst the Chaos

One of the most profound challenges of becoming a mother is the gradual loss of our individual identities. The all-consuming nature of caring for our little ones and managing household responsibilities often leaves us feeling invisible, overwhelmed, and disconnected from our former selves. This chapter aims to acknowledge and address the struggles faced by moms who have found themselves caught in the vortex of motherhood, particularly those who stay at home while their partners assume the role of primary breadwinners. I want every mom to know that they are seen, understood, and that there is hope for reclaiming their identity and finding a sense of fulfillment beyond the roles of caregiver and homemaker.

The Loss of Identity

Becoming a mom can be both rewarding and challenging, but it can also lead to a profound sense of losing oneself. Many women find themselves consumed by the endless cycle of baby and child-related responsibilities, leaving little time for personal growth and self-expression. This struggle is even more pronounced for moms who stay at home, as the primary focus often becomes the well-being of the children and the upkeep of the household. Some of those struggles include:

1. Feeling Unseen and Undervalued: It's common for

mothers to feel unnoticed or underappreciated, as their contributions to the family may not always be recognized. This can lead to a sense of diminished self-worth and a longing to be seen and acknowledged for who they are beyond their roles as mothers and homemakers.

2. Balancing Roles and Expectations: Navigating the roles of caregiver, partner, and individual can be a delicate balancing act. It becomes especially challenging for moms who have previously pursued careers or have higher education degrees, as they may feel a sense of disconnection from their pre-motherhood identities.

Embracing Personal Growth and Nurturing Relationships

While the struggle to regain a sense of identity and balance is real, it is essential to recognize that personal growth and fulfillment are not mutually exclusive from motherhood. Here, we will explore strategies to help moms navigate these challenges and cultivate personal growth.

1. Carving Out Time for Self-Exploration: Allocating dedicated time for personal pursuits and self-exploration is crucial. Whether it's pursuing hobbies, furthering education, or engaging in activities that ignite passion and creativity, these moments of self-discovery can reignite a sense of purpose and individuality.

2. Open Communication and Mutual Support: Honest and open communication with your partner about your personal struggles, aspirations, and need for support is essential. By sharing your feelings and experiences, you can foster a deeper understanding and work together

to create an environment that supports your personal growth.

3. Establishing Boundaries and Sharing Responsibilities: Setting boundaries and communicating your needs regarding household responsibilities can help alleviate feelings of being overwhelmed or taken for granted. Working together with your partner to create a balanced division of tasks can foster a more equitable and supportive environment.

Dear moms, I see you

To all the moms who feel unseen, overwhelmed, or trapped in the roles of caregiver and homemaker, please know that you are not alone. The struggle to find your place and reclaim your identity is a journey that many moms have embarked upon. By acknowledging these challenges and implementing strategies for personal growth, self-expression, and open communication within your relationships, you can gradually rediscover your sense of self and create a life that encompasses both fulfilling motherhood and personal fulfillment. Remember, you are worthy of recognition, support, and the opportunity to nurture your own growth. Embrace this journey with hope, resilience, and the belief that one day, you will find the balance and fulfillment you seek.

Recognizing working moms

Additionally, it's important to acknowledge that working moms face their own set of challenges, albeit in a different context. Balancing the demands of motherhood with professional responsibilities can create a unique struggle. Working moms may experience guilt, burnout, and the constant pressure to excel in both roles. The need for constant reminders and self-care remains just as vital for working moms as they navigate the complexities of their dual roles. By embracing repetition and prioritizing self-care, working moms can find the strength to set boundaries, seek support, and maintain their mental health amidst the juggling act of career and motherhood. Remember, whether you're a stay-at-home mom or a working mom, your well-being matters, and carving out time for self-care is essential for your overall happiness and fulfillment.

Chapter 3

The Power of Boundaries:
Respecting Yourself and Others

Maintaining healthy boundaries is crucial for our overall well-being, especially as mothers who juggle numerous responsibilities and relationships. In this chapter, we will explore the significance of boundaries in various aspects of our lives, including our relationships with our spouse, parents, family, and friends. We will discuss how setting and enforcing boundaries can help us find balance and protect our mind, body, and spirit from toxic energy and situations. Additionally, we will provide guidance in recognizing the need for boundaries and offer practical suggestions for addressing them, particularly when it comes to navigating boundaries within marital relationships.

The Importance of Boundaries
for Total Well-being

Establishing and maintaining boundaries is an essential aspect of self-care and ensuring our total well-being. Boundaries act as protective shields, safeguarding our mental, emotional, and physical health. Here, we will delve into the reasons why boundaries are vital and explore their impact on different areas of our lives.

1. Preserving Mental and Emotional Health: Boundaries enable us to create a safe and nurturing space for our minds and emotions. They prevent the infiltration of toxic energy and allow us to prioritize our mental and

emotional well-being.

2. Fostering Healthy Relationships: Boundaries are the cornerstone of healthy relationships. They promote mutual respect, clear communication, and an equitable balance of needs and responsibilities. Setting boundaries can strengthen our connections with loved ones and create a harmonious environment.

Why we need boundaries

Recognizing when boundaries need to be established or reinforced is crucial. It requires self-awareness, active observation of our feelings and responses, and the courage to advocate for our well-being. Here, we will discuss strategies for recognizing the need for boundaries and provide practical suggestions for addressing them.

1. Paying Attention to Your Feelings: Tuning in to your emotions and physical sensations can help you recognize situations or individuals that drain your energy or trigger negative emotions. If you consistently feel anxious, stressed, or uncomfortable in certain relationships or circumstances, it may be an indication that boundaries need to be set.

2. Communicating Your Boundaries: Effective communication is key when it comes to establishing boundaries. Clearly and assertively express your needs, concerns, and limits to the relevant individuals. Use "I" statements to express how their actions or behaviors impact you and what you need from them moving forward.

3. Setting Consequences and Enforcing Boundaries: Boundaries only hold power when they are backed by consequences. Clearly communicate the consequences if your boundaries are not respected and be prepared to

follow through with appropriate actions. Consistency is key in enforcing boundaries.

4. Seek Support and Professional Help: If you find it challenging to address boundaries, particularly within your marital relationship, consider seeking support from trusted friends, family members, or professional counselors. They can provide guidance, perspective, and tools to navigate these sensitive conversations.

Establishing and maintaining boundaries is essential for nurturing your total well-being. By recognizing the need for boundaries, effectively communicating your needs, and enforcing them with consistency, you create an environment that protects your mind, body, and spirit. Remember, you have the right to set boundaries that promote your well-being and support healthy relationships. Embrace the power of boundaries, cultivate self-awareness, and create a life that is filled with positive energy and balanced relationships.

Boundaries within a Marriage

Boundaries within a marital relationship play a crucial role in fostering trust, self-respect, and mutual respect between partners. Respecting each other's privacy from the beginning sets the foundation for a healthy and secure relationship. Here, we will further explore why boundaries with spouses are essential and how they contribute to building trust and cultivating self-respect.

1. Fostering Trust: Trust is the cornerstone of any successful relationship. By setting boundaries that respect each other's privacy and personal space, you establish an atmosphere of trust. When spouses feel confident that their privacy will be respected, they are more likely to open up, be vulnerable, and share their thoughts and feelings freely. Trust allows partners

to feel secure and supported, strengthening the bond between them.

2. Promoting Self-Respect: Boundaries with spouses are not only about protecting individual privacy but also about cultivating self-respect. Respecting your own boundaries and communicating them to your partner sends a powerful message that you value and prioritize your own well-being. This self-respect sets the stage for your partner to also value and respect your needs, boundaries, and individuality.

3. Encouraging Respect for Each Other: Boundaries create a framework for mutual respect within a relationship. When both partners establish and honor their boundaries, it demonstrates a deep respect for each other's autonomy, personal choices, and individuality. Respecting boundaries fosters an environment where each person feels seen, heard, and acknowledged for who they are, strengthening the foundation of the relationship.

4. Reducing Jealousy and Insecurity: Establishing healthy boundaries early on in a relationship can help alleviate feelings of jealousy and insecurity. By respecting each other's privacy, personal interests, and friendships outside the relationship, spouses can cultivate a sense of security and reduce the potential for jealousy to arise. Boundaries create a space for trust to flourish, reducing the need for unnecessary suspicion or possessiveness.

5. Enhancing Communication and Intimacy: Healthy boundaries encourage open and honest communication between spouses. By respecting each other's boundaries, partners create an environment where they feel safe to express their needs, desires, and concerns without fear of judgment or intrusion. This open communication fosters intimacy and strengthens the emotional connection between partners.

In summary, establishing and respecting boundaries within a marital relationship is essential for building trust, cultivating self-respect, and fostering mutual respect between spouses. By honoring each other's privacy, individuality, and personal space, spouses create a foundation of trust that allows for open communication, reduces jealousy and insecurity, and enhances the overall quality of the relationship. Prioritizing boundaries within the marital context contributes to a healthy and fulfilling partnership.

How boundaries impact parenting and communication

The establishment and maintenance of boundaries within a marital relationship not only have a positive impact on the partnership itself but also extend to better parenting and communication within the family dynamic. Here's how:

1. Role Modeling Healthy Relationships: When spouses demonstrate mutual respect, trust, and effective communication through boundary-setting, they serve as positive role models for their children. Children learn about healthy relationships by observing their parents' interactions. By witnessing respectful boundaries, children understand the importance of individual autonomy, mutual respect, and open communication, which they can apply in their own relationships and interactions.

2. Enhanced Parenting Collaboration: Clear and respected boundaries between spouses facilitate effective parenting collaboration. When both parents have a mutual understanding of each other's roles, responsibilities, and limits, they can work together harmoniously to raise their children. Boundaries ensure

that each parent has the space and opportunity to contribute, make decisions, and provide guidance, leading to a more cohesive and balanced parenting approach.

3. Improved Communication with Children: Setting and respecting boundaries within the marital relationship fosters better communication skills that can be applied to interactions with children. Effective communication involves active listening, expressing needs and concerns, and respecting individual boundaries. Parents who have honed their communication skills are better equipped to understand their children's perspectives, address their needs, and foster a healthy parent-child relationship.

4. Emotional Well-being and Stability: Boundaries contribute to emotional well-being and stability within the family unit. When parents establish and respect each other's boundaries, it creates a sense of security, predictability, and consistency for both parents and children. This stable environment promotes emotional well-being, reduces stress and conflict, and allows for the development of healthy coping mechanisms for the entire family.

5. Teaching Consent and Respect: By upholding boundaries within the marital relationship, parents teach their children valuable lessons about consent and respect. Children learn that their parents' boundaries are to be respected, just as they should respect the boundaries of others. This understanding of personal boundaries lays the foundation for healthy interpersonal relationships and helps children develop empathy, understanding, and consideration for others.

In conclusion, the establishment of boundaries within a marital relationship has a profound impact on parenting and communication within the family. By role modeling healthy relationships, enhancing parenting collaboration, improving communication with children, promoting emotional well-being, and teaching consent and respect, parents create an environment that fosters positive interactions and contributes to the overall well-being of the family unit.

Chapter 4

Seeking Help: Overcoming the Stigma of Mental Health Support

As a mom, your days are filled with a multitude of responsibilities and challenges, making it all too easy for anxiety to creep in and take hold. While it's natural to experience occasional worry and stress, chronic anxiety can have a significant impact on your overall well-being. In this chapter, we will explore the common signs of anxiety that often go unnoticed in women, discuss effective coping skills to overcome anxiety, emphasize the importance of managing anxiety daily for better health, and provide guidance on when it may be time to seek professional help.

Recognizing Anxiety Signs Often Ignored

Anxiety can manifest differently in women compared to men, often leading to these signs being overlooked. By understanding and acknowledging these common indicators, you can take proactive steps to manage your anxiety effectively. Here are five signs that commonly go unnoticed:

1. Physical Symptoms: Anxiety often presents itself through physical manifestations such as headaches, muscle tension, stomachaches, and fatigue. These physical signs can easily be attributed to other causes, making it crucial to recognize them as potential anxiety-related symptoms.

2. Persistent Worry: Excessive worrying about everyday situations, upcoming events, or even trivial matters can be a sign of anxiety. Many women dismiss this persistent worry as normal, but if it starts interfering with your daily life, it's time to address it.

3. Racing Thoughts: An anxious mind is often plagued by a constant stream of racing thoughts, making it difficult to focus or relax. Recognizing this symptom can help you understand when anxiety is at play.

4. Irritability and Restlessness: Heightened irritability, restlessness, and an inability to relax are frequently associated with anxiety. These emotions might be mistakenly attributed to stressors in your life, but it's essential to consider anxiety as a possible underlying cause.

5. Avoidance Behavior: Anxiety can lead to avoidance behavior, where you actively try to escape or avoid situations that trigger anxious feelings. This may include social gatherings, public speaking, or even leaving the house altogether. Identifying such avoidance patterns is crucial to addressing anxiety effectively.

Overcoming Anxiety with Coping Skills

Managing anxiety requires a multifaceted approach that combines self-care, lifestyle changes, and practical coping skills. Here are five simple yet effective strategies to help you overcome anxiety:

1. Deep Breathing and Meditation: Practice deep breathing exercises and incorporate meditation into your daily routine. These techniques can help calm your mind,

reduce stress, and alleviate anxiety symptoms.

2. Regular Exercise: Engaging in physical activity releases endorphins, the body's natural mood boosters. Regular exercise not only improves your physical health but also helps regulate your emotions and reduce anxiety.

3. Prioritize Self-Care: Carve out time for self-care activities that bring you joy and relaxation. Whether it's reading a book, taking a bath, or pursuing a hobby, self-care is essential for reducing anxiety and recharging your mental and emotional energy.

4. Cognitive Behavioral Therapy (CBT) Techniques: CBT is an evidence-based therapeutic approach that focuses on identifying and challenging negative thought patterns. Learning and practicing CBT techniques can help reframe your thoughts and reduce anxiety.

5. Establish Supportive Relationships: Surround yourself with a strong support system of friends, family, or fellow moms who understand your experiences. Sharing your thoughts and feelings with trusted individuals can provide comfort and a sense of belonging, which can significantly alleviate anxiety.

The Importance of Seeking Professional Help

While self-help strategies can be effective for managing anxiety, there may come a time when professional intervention becomes necessary. It's crucial to recognize when seeking help from a therapist or psychiatrist is the right step. Consider the following scenarios:

1. Prolonged or Intense Symptoms: If your anxiety symptoms persist for an extended period or significantly interfere with your daily life, it's

important to seek professional guidance.

2. Difficulty Functioning: When anxiety starts impacting your ability to perform essential tasks, maintain relationships, or take care of yourself and your family, professional help is essential.
3. Self-Harm or Suicidal Thoughts: If you experience thoughts of self-harm or suicide, it is imperative to seek immediate professional assistance by contacting a mental health hotline or visiting the nearest emergency room.

Medication as an Option

In some cases, natural coping strategies might not provide sufficient relief from anxiety symptoms. Medications can be a valuable tool to manage anxiety when other methods prove inadequate. A psychiatrist or medical professional can prescribe medications such as anti-anxiety medications or selective serotonin reuptake inhibitors (SSRIs) to help regulate brain chemistry and alleviate symptoms. It is important to discuss potential benefits, risks, and side effects of medications with your healthcare provider.

Managing anxiety is a journey that requires commitment and self-awareness. By recognizing the common signs of anxiety, utilizing effective coping skills, and knowing when to seek professional help, you can take charge of your mental well-being. In the next chapter, we will briefly explore another critical topic: postpartum depression, anxiety, OCD and psychosis. We will discuss some of the signs and symptoms, how to overcome it, and the importance of seeking help when necessary. Remember, taking care of your mental health is an act of self-love and empowerment that will positively impact not only you but also those around you.

Chapter 5

Postpartum: Unveiling the Volcano of Emotions and Recognizing Symptoms

The postpartum period can be an emotional roller coaster, with intense feelings and experiences that may catch new mothers off guard. For some, these emotions may be more than just "baby blues" and could indicate a more significant condition known as postpartum depression (PPD). In this chapter, we will delve into the complexities of postpartum mental health, exploring the differences between PPD, postpartum anxiety, postpartum OCD, and postpartum psychosis. We will also discuss the importance of recognizing and seeking treatment for these conditions, highlighting the potential consequences of leaving them untreated. Finally, we will explore the prognosis of postpartum mental health disorders and the benefits of therapy and medication as effective treatment options.

Understanding Postpartum Mental Health Disorders

1. Differentiating "Baby Blues" from PPD: "Baby blues" are common and temporary mood swings experienced by many new mothers, typically resolving within two weeks. However, if these symptoms persist for longer than two weeks or intensify, it may indicate the presence of postpartum depression.
2. Postpartum Depression (PPD): PPD is a more severe

and longer-lasting condition that affects approximately 10-20% of new mothers. It is characterized by persistent feelings of sadness, loss of interest or pleasure, changes in appetite and sleep patterns, irritability, fatigue, and difficulty bonding with the baby.

3. Postpartum Anxiety and OCD: Postpartum anxiety involves excessive worrying, restlessness, irritability, and intrusive thoughts related to the baby's well-being. Postpartum OCD involves obsessive thoughts and repetitive behaviors, often centered around the baby's safety and health.

4. Postpartum Psychosis: Postpartum psychosis is a rare but serious condition that requires immediate medical attention. It is characterized by hallucinations, delusions, disorientation, and erratic behavior.

The Importance of Seeking Treatment

1. Consequences of Untreated Postpartum Mental Health Disorders: Leaving postpartum mental health disorders untreated can have profound effects on the mother, the baby, and the family as a whole. It can impact the mother's ability to care for herself and the baby, strain relationships, and lead to long-term mental health complications.

2. Seeking Professional Help: Recognizing the symptoms and understanding when it is more than "baby blues" is crucial. If symptoms persist for longer than two weeks or significantly impact daily functioning, it is important to seek professional help from a therapist, psychiatrist, or other mental health providers who specialize in

postpartum mental health.

Treatment Options and Prognosis

1. Therapy: Therapy, such as cognitive-behavioral therapy (CBT), is a highly effective treatment for postpartum mental health disorders. It helps individuals identify and modify negative thought patterns, develop coping skills, and enhance their support systems.
2. Medications: In some cases, medication, such as antidepressants, may be prescribed to alleviate symptoms of postpartum mental health disorders. These medications can help stabilize mood and restore the chemical imbalances that contribute to the conditions.
3. Prognosis and Recovery: With appropriate treatment, the prognosis for postpartum mental health disorders is generally positive. Many women experience significant improvement in their symptoms and go on to lead fulfilling lives as mothers and individuals. Recovery timelines vary, but with therapy and, if necessary, medication, most women can expect gradual improvement within a few months.

Postpartum mental health disorders can be overwhelming and confusing, but they are treatable conditions. Recognizing the signs and seeking help is the first step towards healing. Remember, postpartum mental health disorders are not a life sentence, and with the right support, therapy, and, if necessary, medication, mothers can recover and find joy in their motherhood journey. You are not alone, and there is hope for a brighter future.

Chapter 6

Simple Routines for Overwhelmed Moms: Managing Responsibilities

As a mom, it's easy to become overwhelmed by the countless responsibilities and demands of daily life. However, implementing simple routines and prioritizing self-care can help you regain a sense of balance, reduce stress, and enhance your overall well-being. In this chapter, we will explore practical routines that can help you manage overwhelming responsibilities, including creating a schedule, tackling household tasks, prioritizing self-care, and incorporating outdoor activities to boost your mood and energy.

Creating a Schedule and Managing Household Tasks

1. Establishing a Daily Routine: Creating a daily schedule can provide structure and help you manage your time more effectively. Start by identifying key tasks and responsibilities, such as childcare, work, and household chores. Allocate specific time blocks for each activity to ensure a sense of accomplishment and prevent feeling overwhelmed.

2. Divide and Conquer: Break down household tasks into manageable chunks. Designate specific days for tasks like laundry, cleaning different rooms, and grocery shopping. By focusing on one room or task per day, you can maintain a tidy and organized home without feeling overwhelmed.

3. Prioritizing Tasks: Understand that not everything

needs to be done immediately. Learn to prioritize tasks based on urgency and importance. For example, dishes can wait while you tend to more pressing matters. By setting realistic priorities, you can alleviate unnecessary stress and focus on what truly matters.

Prioritizing Self-Care

1. Fresh Air and Sunlight: Make it a habit to spend time outdoors each day. Fresh air and sunlight provide numerous benefits, including an increase in vitamin D production and a boost in mood and energy levels. Take a walk in nature, sit in the backyard, or simply open a window to let in natural light.
2. Self-Care in the Shower: Showers can be a rejuvenating self-care practice. Consider incorporating aromatherapy by using scented soaps or essential oils. Take a few extra minutes to enjoy the warm water, allowing it to wash away stress and rejuvenate your body and mind.
3. Dress for the Day: It's easy to fall into the trap of staying in pajamas all day when juggling motherhood and responsibilities. However, getting dressed can boost your mood, increase productivity, and provide a sense of normalcy. Put on comfortable yet presentable clothes that make you feel confident and ready to tackle the day.

Empowering Yourself

1. Setting Boundaries: Establish clear boundaries with others to protect your time, energy, and well-being.

Learn to say "NO" when necessary and communicate your needs effectively. Setting boundaries empowers you to prioritize self-care and prevent burnout.

2. Seek Support: Don't hesitate to reach out for support from family, friends, or support groups. Surrounding yourself with a supportive community can provide validation, encouragement, and practical help when needed.

Implementing simple routines and prioritizing self-care are essential tools for managing overwhelming responsibilities as a mom. By creating a schedule, dividing tasks, prioritizing self-care, and empowering yourself through boundaries and seeking support, you can find balance, reduce stress, and nurture your overall well-being. Remember, taking care of yourself is not selfish, it's a vital component of being a present and thriving mom.

The Value of Constant Reminders

When it comes to maintaining healthy mental health and taking care of ourselves, repetition may sound repetitive itself. However, the power of constant reminders cannot be understated. In this chapter, we will explore the importance of embracing repetition as a tool for achieving and sustaining optimal mental health. By consistently reminding ourselves of self-care practices, boundaries, and the significance of prioritizing our well-being, we can create lasting positive change and cultivate a healthier version of ourselves.

1. Reinforcing Healthy Habits: Repetition serves as a

reinforcement mechanism for healthy habits. By consistently reminding ourselves of the importance of self-care, setting boundaries, and prioritizing mental health, we reinforce these behaviors in our daily lives. Over time, these habits become ingrained, making it easier to maintain a balanced and healthy lifestyle.

2. Overcoming Negative Self-Talk: Repetition helps counteract negative self-talk and self-sabotaging beliefs. By repeatedly reminding ourselves of positive affirmations, self-compassion, and our inherent worth, we can challenge and reframe negative thoughts. This practice builds resilience, self-esteem, and a healthier mindset.

3. Building Consistency: Constant reminders create a sense of consistency and routine in our lives. They serve as gentle nudges to stay on track, ensuring that self-care practices, boundaries, and other healthy habits remain a regular part of our daily lives. Consistency is key to long-term success and positive change.

Utilizing Reminders for Mental Health and Self-Care

1. Visual Cues: Surround yourself with visual cues that serve as reminders. Place sticky notes with affirmations, self-care reminders, or boundary-setting prompts in visible locations such as your bathroom mirror, workspace, or refrigerator. These visual cues serve as gentle reminders to prioritize your mental health and well-being throughout the day.

2. Digital Reminders: Leverage the power of technology by setting up digital reminders on your phone or computer. Use calendar alerts, task management apps, or even dedicated reminder apps to prompt you to engage in

self-care activities, take breaks, or practice mindfulness. These reminders can help you stay accountable and maintain consistency.

3. Supportive Networks: Build a supportive network of family, friends, or online communities who share your commitment to mental health and self-care. Engage in regular check-ins, discussions, or reminders with these individuals to reinforce positive habits, share resources, and hold each other accountable.

Embracing the Journey

1. Embracing Imperfection: Remember that embracing repetition does not mean striving for perfection. It's natural to stumble or have setbacks along the way. Allow yourself grace and compassion as you navigate the path to better mental health and self-care. Each day is an opportunity for growth and improvement.
2. Celebrating Progress: Take time to acknowledge and celebrate the progress you make along the journey. Recognize the positive changes you have implemented, no matter how small. Celebrating milestones and achievements reinforces the importance of constant reminders and encourages continued dedication to your well-being.

While repetition may sound redundant, it is through constant reminders that we solidify healthy mental health practices and self-care habits. Embracing repetition allows us to reinforce positive behaviors, challenge negative thought patterns, and build consistency. By utilizing visual cues, digital reminders, and supportive networks, we can cultivate a healthier mindset and prioritize our well-being. Embrace the journey, celebrate progress, and remind yourself daily that you are worthy of a healthy and fulfilling life.

Chapter 7

Building your Village: Finding Support in Others

Motherhood can sometimes feel like a solitary journey, but it doesn't have to be. Building a supportive network, or "finding your village," is crucial for your well-being as a mom. In this chapter, we will explore the significance of finding your village, how it can positively impact your mental health, and practical steps to cultivate a strong support system. By surrounding yourself with understanding and empathetic individuals, you can navigate the challenges of motherhood with greater resilience, connection, and a sense of belonging.

Understanding the Power of Community

1. Emotional Support: Motherhood can be emotionally demanding, and having a supportive network provides a safe space to share your joys, concerns, and frustrations. Your village offers a listening ear, empathy, and understanding, reminding you that you're not alone in your experiences.
2. Validation and Empowerment: Your village serves as a source of validation, reminding you that your feelings and experiences as a mom are valid. They empower you to trust your instincts, make decisions confidently, and embrace your unique journey.
3. Shared Wisdom and Resources: Being part of a community allows you to tap into a wealth of knowledge and resources. Your village members can provide

valuable insights, practical tips, and recommendations on various aspects of motherhood, from childcare to self-care practices.

Cultivating Your Village

1. Reach Out to Other Moms: Start by connecting with other moms in your local community, online forums, or social media groups. Attend parent support groups, playgroups, or community events specifically tailored for moms. These platforms provide opportunities to meet like-minded individuals who share similar experiences and can become part of your village.
2. Nurture Authentic Relationships: Focus on building genuine connections with other moms. Look for individuals who are non-judgmental, supportive, and share similar values and interests. Invest time and effort in cultivating these relationships, both in-person and online, to foster a sense of camaraderie and trust.
3. Expand Your Network: Don't limit your village to just moms. Include supportive family members, close friends, neighbors, and even professionals such as therapists or counselors who can provide additional guidance and support. Remember, your village can be diverse and multidimensional.

Nurturing Your Village

1. Regular Check-Ins: Maintain regular communication with members of your village. Check in on each other's well-being, share updates, and offer support when needed. Establishing a consistent line of communication fosters a sense of connectedness and

solidarity.

2. Collaborative Activities: Plan and engage in activities together, such as playdates, outings, or even virtual meet-ups. These shared experiences not only create lasting memories but also strengthen the bonds within your village.

3. Give and Receive Support: Remember that supporting others is a two-way street. Offer your help, advice, and encouragement to fellow moms, but also be open to receiving support when you need it. Embrace the reciprocity within your village, as everyone benefits from the give-and-take dynamics.

Finding your village is not just about building a support network; it's about cultivating a sense of belonging, understanding, and empowerment. Surrounding yourself with compassionate and like-minded individuals who share in the joys and challenges of motherhood can provide invaluable emotional support, validation, and shared wisdom. Nurturing your village requires effort, but the rewards are immeasurable. Remember, you are not alone on this journey. Your village stands beside you, empowering you to embrace motherhood with strength, resilience, and a sense of community.

Chapter 8

Strengthening Relationships: Nurturing Bonds with Partners and Friends

If the idea of building a support network or finding your village feels daunting, especially if you're not naturally a people person, it's time to step out of your comfort zone. While it may feel challenging at first, embracing connections and seeking out a supportive community can significantly enhance your well-being as a mom. In this chapter, we will explore practical strategies to help you navigate social interactions, overcome hesitations, and find your village, even if you consider yourself an introvert or struggle with socializing.

Embracing Social Interactions

1. Start Small: Begin by taking small steps outside your comfort zone. Attend local community events, join online forums, or engage in activities that align with your interests. Gradually expose yourself to social interactions, allowing yourself to become more comfortable and confident over time.
2. Be Open and Approachable: Project an open and approachable demeanor when engaging with others. Smile, maintain eye contact, and show genuine interest in conversations. Simple gestures like these can make it easier for others to approach you, fostering connections and potential friendships.
3. Practice Active Listening: Cultivate active listening skills

to show genuine interest in others. By truly listening and engaging in meaningful conversations, you can establish deeper connections. Ask open-ended questions and be present in the moment to foster meaningful interactions.

Seeking Out Supportive Communities

1. Join Online Communities: If in-person interactions feel overwhelming, consider joining online communities focused on motherhood, parenting, or specific interests. These virtual spaces provide an opportunity to connect with like-minded individuals, share experiences, and seek support from the comfort of your own home.
2. Attend Support Groups or Workshops: Seek out local support groups or workshops tailored to moms. These gatherings often provide a safe and understanding environment where you can connect with others who share similar experiences. This shared sense of understanding can help break down barriers and form authentic connections.
3. Volunteer or Engage in Community Activities: Participating in volunteer work or community activities allows you to contribute to a cause while also meeting new people. By engaging in activities aligned with your values and passions, you increase the likelihood of connecting with individuals who share similar interests.

Embracing Growth and
Self-Reflection

1. Challenge Negative Thoughts: Recognize and challenge

any negative thoughts or self-doubt that may arise when stepping out of your comfort zone. Remind yourself that growth and connection often occur outside of familiar territory, and embrace the possibility of positive experiences.

2. Practice Self-Care: Prioritize self-care to ensure you have the emotional resilience to navigate social interactions. Taking care of your physical and mental well-being will boost your confidence and provide a solid foundation as you step out of your comfort zone.

3. Embrace Authenticity: Remember that authenticity is key when seeking meaningful connections. Be true to yourself, embrace your unique qualities, and trust that the right people will be drawn to your genuine self.

Stepping out of your comfort zone is an essential step in finding your village and building a supportive network. Embracing social interactions, seeking out supportive communities, and challenging negative thoughts are all part of the process. By being open, engaging in active listening, and practicing self-care, you can gradually overcome hesitations and find your tribe. Remember, the journey to finding your village may feel uncomfortable at times, but the connections and support you gain along the way are worth the effort. Embrace the growth, nurture authentic relationships, and watch as your village becomes a source of strength, understanding, and empowerment in your motherhood journey.

Nurturing Friendships: The Importance of Prioritizing Connections

In the whirlwind of motherhood, it's easy to let friendships take a backseat. However, maintaining and nurturing friendships is vital for your well-being as a mom. In this chapter, we'll delve into why it's important not to push away your friends and how prioritizing connections can enrich your life. We'll explore practical strategies to ensure that you don't wait for years to enjoy a girls' night out, a trip, or a simple lunch with your friends. By investing in your friendships, you create a support system that adds joy, understanding, and a sense of balance to your motherhood journey.

The Value of Friendship

1. Emotional Support: Friends provide a unique level of emotional support that complements the support you receive from family and partners. They offer a listening ear, empathy, and a fresh perspective, helping you navigate the challenges of motherhood with greater resilience.
2. Identity Beyond Motherhood: Maintaining friendships allows you to retain a sense of identity beyond your role as a mom. Connecting with friends who know you beyond your parenting role can help you stay connected to your passions, interests, and personal growth.
3. Laughter and Joy: Friends bring laughter, humor, and a sense of lightness into your life. Spending time with friends allows you to let loose, enjoy moments of pure joy, and temporarily escape the responsibilities and demands of motherhood.

Prioritizing Friendships

1. Make Time for Regular Gatherings: Don't wait for years to reconnect with your friends. Prioritize regular gatherings, whether it's a monthly girls' night out, a quarterly trip, or a weekly coffee date. Set aside specific

times in your calendar to ensure you make space for these cherished moments.

2. Embrace Technology: Use technology to stay connected with friends, even when physically apart. Schedule virtual hangouts, video calls, or group chats to bridge the distance and maintain a sense of togetherness.

3. Plan Mom-Friendly Activities: Recognize the challenges of juggling motherhood responsibilities and plan activities that accommodate everyone's needs. Explore kid-friendly venues, involve your friends' children in playdates, or plan outings where moms can bond while also tending to their kids' needs.

Communication and Openness

1. Share Your Needs: Communicate openly with your friends about your desire to nurture the friendship and spend quality time together. Express your needs for connection, support, and shared experiences. By voicing your desires, you can work together to find solutions that accommodate everyone's schedules and priorities.

2. Be Present and Engaged: When you're with your friends, be fully present and engaged. Put away distractions, listen actively, and show genuine interest in their lives. Make the most of the time you have together by fostering meaningful connections.

3. Support and Celebrate Each Other: Celebrate your friends' milestones, successes, and joys. Offer support during challenging times and be a source of encouragement. By nurturing a supportive and uplifting environment, your friendships will flourish.

Pushing away your friends can lead to a sense of isolation and a missed opportunity for valuable connections. By prioritizing friendships, you enrich your life as a mom.

Whether it's through regular gatherings, embracing technology, or open communication, investing in your friendships allows you to access emotional support, maintain a sense of identity, and experience joy and laughter. Remember, true friendships withstand the test of time, distance, and the demands of motherhood. So, don't wait for years to reconnect with your friends, prioritize those connections and enjoy the fulfilling journey of friendship alongside your role as a mom.

Chapter 9

Finding Yourself: Embracing Your Worth Beyond Motherhood

As a mom, it's natural for your world to revolve around your spouse and children. However, it's crucial to remember that finding yourself and embracing your worth extends beyond your role as a caregiver. In this chapter, we will explore the importance of prioritizing your own needs, nurturing your personal growth, and reclaiming your identity outside of motherhood. By recognizing your inherent value and investing in your own well-being, you can lead a more fulfilled and balanced life.

Prioritizing Self-Care

1. Self-Care as a Foundation: Self-care is not selfish; it's a necessary foundation for your well-being. Prioritize activities that rejuvenate and nourish your mind, body, and soul. Set aside time each day for activities that bring you joy, whether it's reading, practicing yoga, painting, or simply enjoying a quiet moment of solitude.
2. Setting Boundaries: Establishing healthy boundaries is essential to ensure that your needs are met. Learn to say no when necessary and communicate your limits to others. By prioritizing your own well-being, you teach others to respect and value your time and energy.
3. Seeking Personal Growth: Embrace opportunities for personal growth and pursue activities that ignite your passions and interests. Engage in hobbies, take up new challenges, or enroll in courses that allow you to expand

your knowledge and skills. This constant growth and learning contribute to your overall sense of fulfillment and self-worth.

Reclaiming Your Identity

1. Explore Your Passions: Rediscover and explore the passions and interests you had before becoming a mom. Engage in activities that bring you joy and remind you of the unique aspects of your identity. Whether it's pursuing a hobby, joining a club, or volunteering for a cause, allow yourself the space to reconnect with your authentic self.
2. Cultivating Independence: While being a mom is a significant part of your life, it's essential to maintain your independence. Foster independence by engaging in activities or outings without your spouse or children. This autonomy reinforces your sense of self and reminds you that you are an individual with your own desires and dreams.
3. Nurture Relationships Beyond Motherhood: While your children and spouse are vital, it's essential to nurture relationships outside of your immediate family. Maintain connections with friends, extended family members, and individuals who provide different perspectives and support. These relationships broaden your social circle and provide a sense of connection beyond your role as a mom.

Embracing a Balanced Life

1. Prioritizing Your Dreams: Don't forget about your dreams and aspirations. Identify your long-term goals

and take small steps towards achieving them. Whether it's pursuing a career, starting a business, or embarking on a personal project, investing in your dreams reaffirms your worth and adds purpose to your life.

2. Finding Moments of Solitude: Carve out moments of solitude to reflect, recharge, and reconnect with yourself. Whether it's a walk in nature, journaling, or meditation, these moments allow you to tune in to your inner voice and gain clarity amidst the busyness of motherhood.

3. Celebrating Your Achievements: Acknowledge and celebrate your achievements, big and small. Recognize your growth as a mother, partner, and individual. Take pride in your accomplishments, and remember that you are deserving of recognition and praise.

Finding yourself beyond motherhood is not a selfish endeavor; it's an essential part of leading a balanced and fulfilling life. By prioritizing self-care, reclaiming your identity, and embracing a balanced approach to life, you reaffirm your worth and create a foundation for personal growth and happiness.

Evolving Dreams: Embracing Change and Rediscovery

1. Embracing Change: It's perfectly normal for your dreams and aspirations to evolve over time, especially as you navigate the transformative journey of motherhood. Embrace the idea that your dreams may shift or take on new forms, and recognize that this is an opportunity for self-discovery and growth.

2. Reflecting on Your Passions: Take time to reflect on what truly brings you joy and fulfillment in the present moment. Explore new interests and engage in activities that spark curiosity and enthusiasm. Allow yourself

the freedom to explore different avenues and be open to discovering passions you may not have previously considered.

3. Redefining Success: As your dreams change, it's important to redefine what success means to you. Instead of solely focusing on external achievements, shift your perspective to embrace personal growth, contentment, and the ability to find joy in the everyday moments of motherhood. Success can be found in the loving relationships you nurture, the resilience you develop, and the happiness you cultivate within yourself.

4. Cultivating Flexibility: As a mom, you understand the importance of adaptability and flexibility. Apply this mindset to your evolving dreams. Embrace the idea that your aspirations may shift in response to the different seasons of motherhood. Be kind to yourself and give yourself permission to explore new paths, even if they deviate from your previous expectations.

5. Seeking Inspiration: If you find yourself unsure of your new dreams or lacking a clear direction, seek inspiration from various sources. Engage in conversations with others, read books or articles on personal development, listen to podcasts or attend workshops that explore topics aligned with your interests. Surrounding yourself with different perspectives and ideas can spark inspiration and guide you towards discovering your renewed dreams.

As your dreams change or evolve, it's an opportunity for self-discovery and embracing the new chapter of your life. Instead of feeling disheartened, approach this phase with curiosity and openness. Reflect on your passions, redefine success on your own terms, and cultivate flexibility in embracing the journey of motherhood. Remember, your dreams may change, but your worth and potential for growth remain constant. Trust yourself, be patient, and allow the process of rediscovery to unfold naturally.

Chapter 10

The Importance of Positive Affirmations and Daily Gratitude

In the midst of the challenges and responsibilities of motherhood, it's important to cultivate a positive mindset and find moments of gratitude. In this chapter, we will explore the transformative power of positive affirmations and daily gratitude practices. By incorporating these practices into your daily routine, you can shift your perspective, enhance your well-being, and foster a greater sense of contentment and joy.

Positive Affirmations

1. Understanding Affirmations: Positive affirmations are powerful statements that reflect your desired state of being or mindset. They can help reframe negative self-talk, overcome self-doubt, and cultivate a more positive and empowered outlook on life. By repeating affirmations, you can rewire your subconscious mind and reinforce positive beliefs about yourself.

2. Creating Personalized Affirmations: Tailor affirmations to your specific needs and aspirations. Identify areas of self-improvement or challenges you want to overcome and craft affirmations that address those aspects. For example, if you struggle with self-confidence, affirmations like "I am confident and capable" or "I embrace my unique strengths" can be powerful reminders of your inherent worth.

3. Incorporating Affirmations into Daily Life: Integrate

affirmations into your daily routine. Repeat them during your morning rituals, write them in a journal, display them in visible places around your home, or use them as mantras during meditation or moments of self-reflection. Consistency is key in harnessing the transformative power of affirmations.

Daily Gratitude Practices

1. Recognizing the Benefits of Gratitude: Cultivating a daily gratitude practice helps shift your focus towards the positive aspects of your life. It enhances your overall well-being, reduces stress, and promotes a more optimistic outlook. Gratitude allows you to appreciate the present moment and find joy in even the smallest of things.

2. Keeping a Gratitude Journal: Set aside a few minutes each day to reflect on and write down things you are grateful for. It could be as simple as the laughter of your children, a warm cup of tea, or a supportive friend. Writing them down helps solidify the positive experiences and encourages a mindset of gratitude.

3. Expressing Gratitude to Others: Extend gratitude beyond yourself by expressing appreciation to the people in your life. Write heartfelt notes, have meaningful conversations, or perform acts of kindness to show your gratitude. Cultivating a culture of gratitude strengthens your relationships and fosters a sense of connection and support.

Integrating Positive Affirmations and Gratitude

1. Morning Rituals: Start your day by setting positive

intentions through affirmations. Combine this with a moment of gratitude, reflecting on three things you are grateful for. This combination sets a positive tone for the day ahead and helps you approach challenges with a more resilient and grateful mindset.

2. Mindful Moments: Throughout the day, pause and take mindful moments to affirm positive beliefs about yourself and express gratitude for the present moment. These brief pauses can ground you, provide clarity, and foster a sense of appreciation for the blessings in your life.

3. Bedtime Reflections: Before you sleep, reflect on the day and identify moments of gratitude. Acknowledge your accomplishments, however small they may be, and recite affirmations that promote self-compassion and positivity. This practice helps you end the day on a positive note and promotes a restful and rejuvenating sleep.

Positive affirmations and daily gratitude practices have the power to transform your mindset and elevate your well-being as a mom. By incorporating these practices into your daily routine, you can shift your perspective, cultivate self-compassion, and find joy in the present moment. Embrace the power of positive affirmations and gratitude, and watch as they enhance your overall happiness, resilience, and gratitude for the journey of motherhood.

53

Conclusion

Embracing the Journey
of Motherhood

Congratulations, dear mom, on reaching the end of this book! You have embarked on a remarkable journey, one filled with joy, challenges, and moments of profound transformation. Throughout these chapters, we have explored a wide range of topics aimed at supporting your well-being, managing anxiety, nurturing relationships, and rediscovering your authentic self.

Remember, motherhood is not meant to be a solitary endeavor. It is a shared experience, and you are not alone. Whether you are a new mom, a seasoned parent, a working mom, or a stay-at-home mom, the struggles and triumphs you face are shared by many. It is within this collective understanding that we find strength, encouragement, and support.

As you navigate the joys and complexities of motherhood, always remember to prioritize your own well-being. Self-care is not selfish, it is a necessary foundation for you to show up as the best version of yourself for your children, your spouse, and everyone around you. Take time to nurture your mind, body, and spirit, and don't be afraid to ask for help when you need it.

Managing anxiety is a journey in itself, and recognizing the signs, seeking professional help when necessary, and practicing coping skills can make a tremendous difference in your overall well-being. Remember, you are not defined by your anxiety, and with the right support, it can be managed effectively.

Additionally, we explored the importance of setting boundaries, nurturing relationships, and finding your village. Surrounding yourself with a supportive community is vital to your mental and emotional well-being. Don't be afraid to step out of your comfort zone, reach out to others, and create connections that uplift and inspire you.

Furthermore, we delved into the topic of postpartum experiences and the importance of seeking help when needed. Postpartum depression, anxiety, OCD, and psychosis are real and impactful challenges. If you find yourself experiencing prolonged and distressing symptoms, do not hesitate to seek professional help. Remember, treatment is available, and you deserve support and care.

In the pursuit of finding balance and reclaiming your identity, remember to honor your dreams, passions, and personal growth. Embrace change, redefine success on your own terms, and allow yourself the space to evolve as an individual alongside your role as a mother. You matter, and the world outside of motherhood is filled with possibilities waiting for you to explore.

Lastly, we discussed the power of positive affirmations and daily gratitude practices. Cultivating a positive mindset, reaffirming your worth, and expressing gratitude for the blessings in your life can create a ripple effect of positivity and contentment. Embrace these practices as daily rituals, and watch as they transform your perspective and bring more joy into your life.

Dear mom, as you conclude this book, know that you are seen, heard, and appreciated. The journey of motherhood is a beautiful tapestry of experiences, emotions, and growth. Embrace the challenges, cherish the moments of connection, and honor the incredible woman that you are.

Remember, you are more than a mom, you are a beacon of love, strength, and resilience. Embrace your power, trust your instincts, and continue to nurture your well-being. You have the ability to create a life filled with joy, purpose, and fulfillment. The world is better because you are in it.

Wishing you an abundance of love, joy, and fulfillment on your journey of motherhood and beyond. You are extraordinary.

With heartfelt gratitude,

Aisha Brady, LMSW, PMH

The Mental Health Coach For Moms

Resources

Postpartum Support International (PSI)

- o Website: www.postpartum.net
- o Helpline: 1-800-944-4773

National Alliance on Mental Illness (NAMI)

- o Website: www.nami.org
- o Helpline: 1-800-950-NAMI (6264)
- o Suicide and Crisis Lifeline: Dial 988

Mindful Mama Podcast with Hunter Clarke-Fields

- o Website: www.mindfulmamamentor.com/podcast

Mother's Mental Health

- Website: https://mothersmentalhealth.org/

Note: Please be aware that the information provided in this book is intended for general informational purposes only. While efforts have been made to ensure the accuracy and relevance of the content, it should not be considered a substitute for professional advice or medical guidance.

Consult with a Medical Professional:

It is strongly recommended that you consult with a qualified medical professional or mental health practitioner for personalized advice and guidance related to your specific situation. Every individual's experiences and circumstances are unique, and a professional can provide a comprehensive assessment and tailored recommendations based on their expertise and knowledge.

While the content in this book is based on the author's experiences and expertise as a counselor, it is important to remember that individual experiences may vary, and what works for one person may not work for another. Therefore, it is essential to consult with a professional who can evaluate your specific needs and provide appropriate guidance.

The author of this book is not responsible for any actions or decisions taken based on the information provided. The reader assumes full responsibility for their own well-being and should exercise caution and discretion when implementing any suggestions or strategies mentioned in this book.

Always prioritize your own health and safety, and seek professional help if you have concerns or questions regarding your mental or physical well-being.

The information provided in this book is for general informational purposes only and is not intended to be a substitute for professional advice. The author and publisher of this book shall not be held liable or responsible for any loss, damage, or injury arising from the use or misuse of the information contained herein.

While every effort has been made to ensure the accuracy and reliability of the information presented, the author and publisher make no representations or warranties of any kind, express or implied, about the completeness, accuracy, reliability, suitability, or availability of the information, products, services, or related graphics contained in this book.

The reader acknowledges that their use of any information or materials provided in this book is at their own risk. It is recommended that readers consult with qualified professionals, such as medical practitioners, mental health experts, or legal advisors, for individualized guidance pertaining to their specific circumstances.

By reading this book, the reader acknowledges and agrees to release, indemnify, and hold harmless the author and publisher from any claims, damages, or losses arising out of or in connection with the use of this ebook.

Please consult a professional or expert in the relevant field for advice and assistance specific to your situation.

www.ingramcontent.com/pod-product-compliance
Lightning Source LLC
Chambersburg PA
CBHW071109260726
48661CB00006B/2547